CAREER AS AN

OSTEOPATHIC PHYSICIAN

DOCTOR OF OSTEOPATHY (DO)

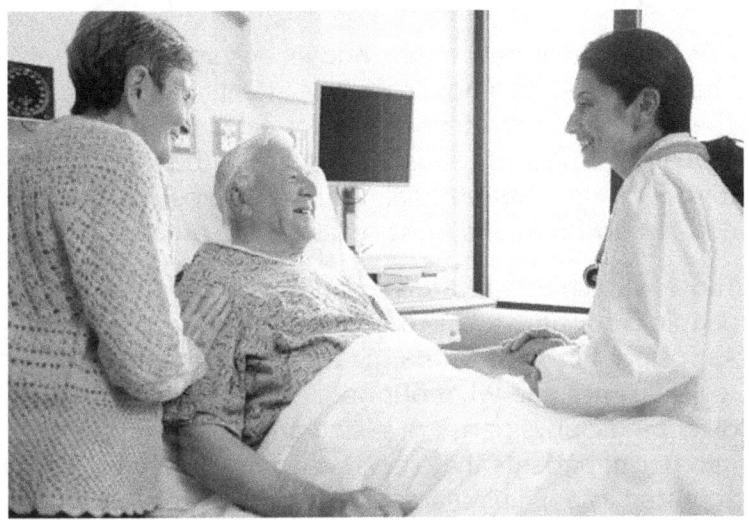

THERE ARE OVER 43,000 OSTEOPATHIC physicians in the United States, providing a system of medical care based on a philosophy that the human body has self-healing abilities. In order to facilitate those abilities, the osteopathic doctor practices a "whole person" approach. While the goal of traditional medical doctors is to treat specific symptoms, osteopathic physicians concentrate on treating the patient as a whole.

It is important to make this distinction. *Osteopaths,* who are trained outside the United States are not physicians. Their practice is limited to non-invasive manual therapies, including touch, physical manipulation, stretching and massage to increase the mobility of joints, to relieve muscle tension, and to help energize the body's own healing mechanisms.

Those trained in the United States are known as *osteopathic physicians* (or Doctors of Osteopathy or DOs), and they practice the entire scope of modern medicine. They receive all the training and provide the same healthcare services as medical doctors (MDs).

DOs understand how all the body's systems are interconnected and how each one affects the others. They are trained to identify and correct structural problems, which can assist the body's natural tendency toward health and self-healing. They also help patients develop attitudes and lifestyles that help prevent disease.

Those who choose a career in osteopathic medicine are people who value taking a holistic approach to healing. As society shifts towards a greater understanding of what makes us sick and what our bodies are capable of, osteopathic physicians are seeing an increase in the number of patients they see. Osteopathy in the US is fully accepted as a mainstream medical career. Today, millions of Americans have chosen this type of individualized, compassionate care, and have made DOs their primary care physicians.

Osteopathic medicine as a profession began in the late 1800s, however, the concept actually dates back much further. The human body's ability to heal itself is more natural than invasive surgery or prescription drugs. Osteopathic physicians employ a simpler way of treating disease and illness than their MD counterparts.

The practice of osteopathy experienced rejection as it officially emerged. It had to fight against the medical establishment in terms of education, licensing, and recognition as its own form of medicine. It was even called a "cult" by the American Medical Association (which has since retracted those words). The field prevailed, thanks in large part to some influential supporters. Perhaps the most famous proponent of osteopathic medicine was Mark Twain, who believed in it so firmly that he publicly spoke about its ability to heal and lobbied for its national acceptance.

In terms of training and education, osteopathic physicians (DOs) are actually indistinguishable from medical doctors (MDs). They are trained in similar schools, go through the same number of years, learn the procedures, and pass the same examinations. They have the same rights and privileges to practice medicine. The difference is in how they choose to treat the patient. When MDs might reach for the prescription pad, a DO might prescribe a change of diet or environment instead.

Like their MD colleagues, DOs can specialize in over a hundred different areas of practice. Because of their total-person philosophy, many gravitate to specialties in primary care fields such as family medicine, pediatrics, obstetrics, and emergency medicine. DOs are also specially trained in manual medicine for treatment of musculoskeletal disorders. This makes them uniquely qualified to specialize in rehabilitation and sports medicine. In fact, many DOs are employed as professional sports and college team physicians.

DOs have an extensive scientific background. They must excel in science classes like biology, chemistry, and anatomy. They learn all of the traditional medical techniques, but they also receive additional training in muscular-skeletal manipulation. They also complete a residency in a specialty.

Osteopathic physicians spend a significant amount of time and money on medical school, dedicating upwards of seven years of their life to study in some cases. As a result, they do have a higher-than-average median salary. Earnings can reach well into the six figures, making it quite an attractive job for compassionate individuals with a love of healing and science.

There is a growing shortage of healthcare professionals in this country. This makes it an ideal time to get into the medical field, particularly the area of osteopathic medicine, which is set to see phenomenal growth throughout this upcoming decade.

WHAT YOU CAN DO NOW

IF YOU ARE INTERESTED IN A CAREER in osteopathic medicine, you can start by taking the right classes in high school. One of the most important classes is biology. The fundamentals of all medicine start in biology. Does your school offer an advanced biology course to earn advanced placement in college? You will definitely want to add this to your class schedule. Explore any classes that will teach you more about the human body, such as the musculoskeletal system, disease and disease prevention, organs and their purpose, and bacteria.

Load up on other science classes as well. Chemistry is particularly important. It lays the foundation for knowledge of prescription medicine and how different chemicals interact with one another and affect the human body. If your school offers health or nutrition classes, these would make a great complement to your scientific background and would help prepare you for a career in osteopathic medicine.

You will need to keep your grades high throughout high school and college in order to qualify for admission to medical school. Good performance on tests and doing extra credit where possible will help ensure that you get into the best school possible.

To learn more about what an osteopath does, you need to see the career from the inside. Ask your guidance counselor to help you arrange a day (or more) of job shadowing. There are DOs practicing everywhere, even in small towns. Most will be willing to invite you into their offices, show you the daily routine, and answer any questions you might have.

HISTORY OF THE PROFESSION

OSTEOPATHIC MEDICINE FIRST emerged as a distinct healthcare profession in the late 1800s in Kirksville, Missouri. The doctor who founded it had the very unique belief that the current way of treating patients was actually causing more harm than good. He knew there was a need for humans to heal themselves instead of relying so heavily on the medical practices that were common then. After all, he reasoned, healing is a natural process of the body. Therefore, on some level, couldn't traditional medicine be considered "unnatural"? Might there be a better way to handle human ailments? With this simple idea, a more holistic approach to medicine was born.

While osteopathic medicine is its own distinctive branch of medicine, it would not exist without the medical foundation on which it stands. For that we have to travel much further back into history. Western medicine as we know it is actually an amalgamation of practices from all across the ancient world.

The ancient Egyptians and Babylonians are thought to have introduced the concepts of diagnosis, prognosis (forecasting recovery), and medical examination to humanity. The Greeks contributed medical ethics to the field of medicine, including the Hippocratic Oath every doctor is required to take to this day.

Beginning in the medieval era, medicine began to experience major advances in surgery. Around the same time, the systematic training of physicians started in Italy in 1220. As time went on, technologies were developed, including the microscope, during the Renaissance. Each of these steps has created the base for modern medicine as we know it today.

In the 19th century, medicine saw the development of the germ theory of disease, the idea that disease is actually caused by nasty little unseen organisms that propagate and multiply. This discovery, which we now consider common sense, actually changed the course of human history. It led directly to the first successful measures that were taken to stop the spread of disease through simple practices, such as hand washing and better public sanitation.

In the mid-20th century, the field of medicine saw many major advances. Antibiotics were introduced and accepted as the cure for many ailments. Technological advancements such as X-rays helped usher in a new age of modern medicine. This is also the time that healthcare became professionalized. For the first time, physicians were encouraged to choose a specialty area instead of being a general practitioner of medicine. Even family doctors were declared specialists, with all the additional education and certifications that implies. The number of specialties and subspecialties for medical doctors grew to 130. The field of osteopathy followed a similar trend, with DOs eventually being able to choose from a list of over 100 specialty areas of practice.

By the end of the 20th century, medicine itself had

become a booming business, responsible for billions of dollars a year in the economy. Amid this explosive growth, traditional medicine had become very dependent on technology. Osteopathy continued on its holistic path, recognizing that long before the introduction of antibiotics, nature provided cures to many ailments such as peppermint for tummy aches and aloe for burns. Long ago, those who prescribed plants as a cure were known as shamans or apothecaries. Today they are much more likely to be herbalists or osteopathic physicians.

Andrew Taylor Still founded the American School of Osteopathy in the 19th century on the basis of healing through work on the musculoskeletal system, surgery, and the occasional well-placed drug. When it first emerged as a profession, osteopathy faced significant scrutiny from the established medical profession, which tried to discredit it. In fact, for the first half of the 20th century, osteopathic medicine was vigorously opposed by the American Medical Association. Physicians licensed as medical doctors were forbidden to even associate with osteopaths.

The battle for regulation and licensing of osteopaths began in the second half of the 20th century. In 1966, Secretary of Defense Robert McNamara allowed osteopaths to practice in medical military services with the same privileges as MDs. Although it appeared to be a win for osteopaths, the battle raged on. In California, Proposition 22 actually eliminated the practice from the state altogether. Those who had obtained their DO license paid a fee to switch it over to an MD. The University of California at Irvine College of Osteopathic Medicine was renamed as the University of California, Irvine School of Medicine. DOs who moved into California were banned from being issued a physician's license, too. The tide began to turn in 1974 when the California Supreme Court ruled that the licensing of DOs must be resumed.

The American Medical Association (AMA) first began to allow qualified osteopathic physicians to become members as well as to participate in internships and residency programs in 1969. However, the American Osteopathic Association rejected this invitation. They felt it was the AMA's attempt to eliminate osteopathic medicine as its own discipline altogether and assimilate it back in with traditional medicine yet again. This was also resolved, and today DOs and MDs are trained and practice alongside one another.

Osteopathic doctors also faced discrimination at the state level in terms of licensing of practice rights. The back and forth battle of DOs versus MDs lasted for much of the 20th century. The final state to allow DOs to practice on the same level as MDs was Nebraska in 1989. Today, the training and practice between DOs and MDs are mostly indistinguishable. Those physicians who have obtained their DO outside of the United States are not allowed to practice here, but DOs who have obtained their license in this country can fully practice in 45 countries and partially practice in many more around the globe.

WHERE DOs WORK

PEOPLE WHO WORK IN THE FIELD OF osteopathic medicine have a few options when it comes to where they work. The first option is to join a hospital as one of its full-time staff doctors. In this scenario, you would be employed by the hospital directly, reporting to a Chief of Staff.

Osteopathic physicians traditionally work 40 hours a week in the standard 9 to 5 timetable. When you work for a private hospital though, you may have less say over what kind of hours you work. As patients have no control over when they get sick, physicians in hospital settings may have to work nights, weekends, and holidays. You may also experience a more complicated rotating schedule, which changes week to week. It could be 9 to 5 one week, overnights the next week, followed by a week off. Being "on call" is also a reality of working for a hospital. Being on call means there will be nights where you do not have to be at the hospital physically, but you will need to be available to come in at a moment's notice if called.

Hospital work settings depend on the size and specialty of the hospital. The typical environment would be brightly lit with easy-to-clean tile or laminate flooring in work areas, and neutral carpets in patient lounges. The wall colors are also muted, to keep the patients calm as they come down the hallways or sit in the rooms. A hospital environment is also quiet with low levels of volume.

In most cases, you would have a private office. This is usually a modest room where you can keep files, have privacy, and rest between seeing patients. There may also be a doctor's lounge, a location similar to a public waiting room, where you can get a cup of coffee or a snack, and take a break between appointments.

Many osteopathic physicians choose to start their own private practice. The biggest advantage to being in private practice is having control over the type of cases you handle and your schedule. Private practice osteopaths traditionally work a set weekly schedule of 9 to 5 or maybe 8 to 4. Nights and weekends are not scheduled, but some physicians give their home phone numbers or cell phones to patients so they can be reached in case of an emergency.

Osteopathic physicians who work in a private practice may be self-employed, working solo as the only physician in an office. Increasingly, however, many are choosing to join a network of other physicians to create a small group practice. Working together this way helps lower costs while increasing the size of the patient base more quickly.

Not all osteopathic doctors work directly with patients. Some are employed by laboratories. Others serve as staff consultants for private companies.

THE WORK YOU WILL DO

THE DAY-TO-DAY WORK DUTIES OF osteopathic physicians depend primarily on their areas of expertise, as well as the environment in which they work. For example, the work of an osteopath who specializes in pediatrics would vary greatly from an osteopath who specializes in oncology. However, the routine is similar for all DOs who work directly with patients.

Whether in a hospital or private practice setting, osteopathic physicians follow the same steps from the patient's diagnosis through recovery. These routine responsibilities include:

- Taking the patient's medical history and asking certain intake questions
- Performing the initial examination
- Making the diagnosis
- Creating an actionable treatment plan
- Setting up a schedule of follow-up appointments
- Prescribing medication when necessary

- Tracking the patient's progress throughout the treatment

- Making referrals to other healthcare professionals when appropriate

- Educating the patient regarding relevant lifestyle choices

- Filling out paperwork and entering computer records

- Intake and Examination

The patient's visit would start with an intake questionnaire and examination. The DO would ask questions about the history of the condition or discomfort as well as detailed questions about the patient's lifestyle and environment. These doctors tend to take more time with their patients, getting to know them on an individual level. Relationship building comes into play here. The root of the problem is often something that runs deeper than a strain of bacteria. The osteopath might seem more like a therapist than a doctor at first, asking the patient probing questions. The answers might uncover a psychological reason behind the physical symptoms. For example, it is well known that stress has an adverse effect on health. Therefore, if a patient comes in reporting frequent infections, the osteopathic physician might start by recommending stress management after learning that the patient has been experiencing a stressful time.

After the initial consultation comes the physical examination. The osteopathic physician might ask the patient to perform simple movements to observe how the patient uses the body. Because DOs are trained in subtle musculoskeletal differences, watching patients move their limbs or something similar can help significantly with a diagnosis. The DO will pay special attention to mobility and posture throughout the visit. The patient may also be asked to take certain physical tests that are designed to demonstrate neurological activity. During the examination, the osteopath will start with the area of discomfort. Unlike a traditional medical doctor, the DO is more concerned with the whole body and how it affects the issue of concern. Therefore, the osteopath may move from place to place on a patient's body, examining the joints, spine, muscles, and tendons. In some cases, blood tests or X-rays may be ordered.

Treatment Plan

Once the physical examination is complete, the osteopathic physician recommends a specialized treatment plan that is highly individualized. In general, the osteopathic physician's approach to healing involves improving the lymphatic, circulatory, and nervous systems so they function at a more efficient level. This may allow the body to heal itself more naturally without the intervention of surgery or prescription drugs. Potential remedies might include stretching to improve blood flow and articulation of the joints, and exercise to energize the muscles.

Osteopaths are best known for working very closely with the musculoskeletal system. This is not surprising since it is one of the founding principles of osteopathy. DOs believe that many health problems can best be solved by gently manipulating tissue, bones, and muscles. They use a variety of hands-on techniques that are designed to reset the body, eliminate inflammation, and restore the body's ability to heal naturally. This might include adjusting limbs, massaging different points, or stretching certain muscles. The goal of this form of manipulative medicine is to alleviate pain, restore motion, encourage the natural tendency of the body to heal itself, and eliminate blockages that would interfere with that healing.

The treatment plan might also include recommendations for lifestyle changes, particularly in the area of diet and nutrition. For example, putting a patient on an elimination diet is quite common. That would involve removing certain foods from a patient's diet and then slowly reintroducing them. The goal is to discover any trigger foods that can be causing inflammation throughout the body, leading to bigger problems. The treatment might also include an element of stress management, which could come in the form of meditation, journaling practices, or regular exercise. In some cases, an osteopathic physician might determine it would be beneficial to work in conjunction with other practitioners in different healthcare specialties, so the body is treated in a more holistic approach.

As licensed physicians, osteopaths have access to prescription pads. They can and do prescribe medication when it is needed, but it is rarely the first order of treatment. Osteopaths can also perform surgery – and they sometimes do. In fact, some DOs choose to specialize in surgery.

Specializations

Just as with medical doctors, osteopathic physicians can choose an area in which to specialize. This significantly affects the work that they do. Most osteopathic physicians, almost 40 percent, choose primary care as their specialty. In fact, this specialty is more popular among DOs than MDs. In addition, there are more than a hundred specialties to choose from in osteopathy, from anesthesiology to urology.

Anesthesiology involves pain management. In a surgery center, that means administering anesthesia to patients before they go under the knife. But DOs, who are always looking at the bigger picture, also assess their patients' pain and develop a plan to manage that pain throughout the entire surgery experience, including pre-surgery, during surgery, and post-surgery. This specialty can also be applied to private practice. In this case, the DO would typically be practicing long-term pain management.

Dermatology is primarily concerned with the skin, hair, and nails. It also covers the treatment of the various mucus membranes of the body. Osteopathic dermatologists regularly examine their patients for abnormalities of the skin, including moles, skin cancer, rashes, and acne. They also treat abnormalities of the hair such as baldness, and problems with the nails. They may also perform minor surgeries like mole or wart removal procedures.

Emergency medicine specialists work in hospital ERs (emergency rooms), handling patients who need immediate assistance because of trauma or a surprising onset of symptoms. This is typically a fast-paced environment, where DOs must prioritize patients based on how urgently they need attention. These DOs order tests, diagnose and treat the patients appropriately, and check in with patients as needed. Shifts can be long and arduous for emergency room doctors. They may also find themselves on call frequently and must be available to head to the hospital at a moment's notice when needed.

Internal medicine is a natural area of interest for osteopaths because, like family/general practice, it deals with every system in the body. Osteopaths who practice internal medicine must be familiar with every organ. These DOs work primarily with adults and treat a wide variety of ailments and issues.

Neurology is concerned with the brain, spinal cord, and nerves. DOs in this specialty treat patients who are experiencing headaches, chronic pain, dizziness, numbness or tingling, unexplained vision problems, seizures, sleep problems, difficulty thinking, or problems with movement. They examine patients, order tests such as brain scans, prescribe medication, and conduct patient follow-up.

Obstetrics and gynecology (OB/GYN) is another favorite among osteopathic physicians. These DOs focus on the health of women's reproductive organs. They analyze a patient's medical history, perform regular check-ups, order and administer appropriate tests for the patient's health, and diagnose and treat problems. They also work very closely with a woman throughout her pregnancy, monitoring the baby's and the mother's health, deliver the baby, and provide post-natal care.

Osteopathic surgery is like any other surgery, performed in an operating room with surgical tools and the latest life-saving equipment. DOs who specialize in surgery often pick a subspecialty area such as thoracic, cardiovascular, or urology. The most common subspecialty is orthopedic surgery because of its close relationship to the foundation of osteopathy – the musculoskeletal system. Orthopedic surgeons work on everything that allows a patient to move: ligaments and tendons, muscles, the skeletal system, and joints. They perform corrective surgery that allows a patient to be more active and regain mobility.

Nuclear medicine DOs utilize radioactive substances to diagnose and treat disease. They employ different tinctures in the body that can localize specific organs or cellular receptors, allowing the osteopath to get a clear picture of the body's processes and determine what is working and what is not. From there they develop a treatment plan for the patient, which may or may not include further radioactive substances. This area of specialty is closely linked to diagnostic radiology.

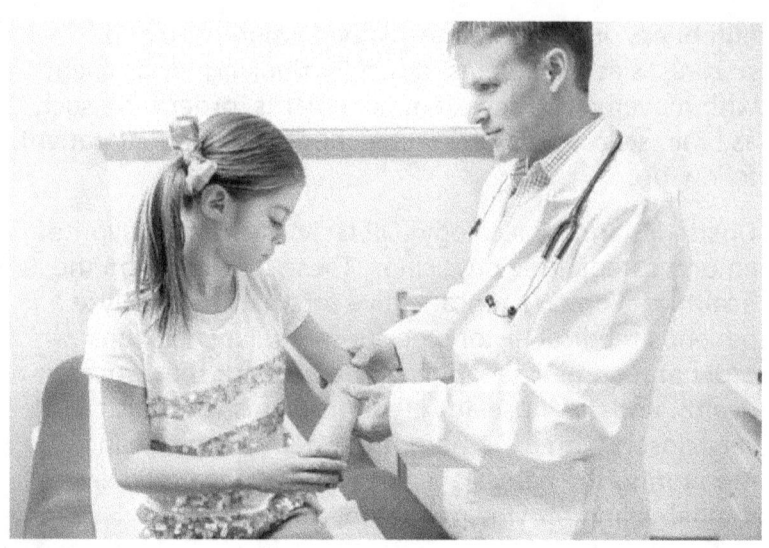

OSTEOPATHIC PHYSICIANS TELL THEIR OWN STORIES

I Am a Locum Tenens DO

"The term *locum tenens* comes from Latin, meaning 'to hold a place.' Its meaning in the medical community is to fill in for other physicians on a temporary basis. I suppose someone decided it's undignified to call a physician a 'temp.' What I like most about this work style is the flexibility of schedule, and the pay. I work only as much as I want, when I want. I take as much time off as I can afford. If a situation doesn't suit me, I pass it back to the company that placed me and they get someone else. I can go anywhere and be on a new job the next day with no repercussions.

The money is amazing. I not only get a great salary, all my expenses are reimbursed – travel, housing, and rental car. I don't even have to pay malpractice insurance, which is a huge burden for any physician in private practice.

My work mostly involves handling the overflow of patients who are the most in need of immediate care. I will put patients in the hospital if needed. It is usually a fast-paced environment so I do a lot of things for myself that most DOs would not do. For example, I read my own x-rays because I know it will be a full day before I get the report back from radiology. I also do my own biopsies, casts, splints, and joint injections.

There really is no typical day. I could be working four 24-hour ER shifts, or I may be seeing 15 to 25 patients a day in a nursing home. I might be doing sports physicals all day, or it could be all OMT (osteopathic manipulative treatment) for everything from migraine headaches to kids with ear infections. Whatever walks through the door, that's what I handle.

My advice to new DOs is don't be quick to take the first job that comes your way. I got stuck in three permanent jobs that were completely unsuitable before I took a step back and took stock of what I really wanted from my career. It would have been much better if I had gone to locums first to find a job that fit me and my personality and needs, so I could walk away easily if I hated it.

You do need to be prepared to travel. Don't limit yourself to a single state license, and do sign up with at least two companies so you will always have work on demand. There are so many jobs out there and such a huge need, particularly in rural areas, that you will always be as busy as you want to be."

I Am an Osteopath in Private Practice

"When I was a teenager I hurt my back playing soccer. It was extremely painful. I could hardly walk it hurt so much. My parents took me to a lot of different people – MDs, chiropractors, physical therapists, and more – but in the end it was an osteopath who helped me. The entire experience made a huge impression and when it came time to choose a career path, osteopathic medicine was all I could think of. Now that I've been practicing for 10 years, I can't imagine doing anything else.

I love my work because it is so diverse. A lot of people think osteopathy is just about bones and maybe put us in the same category as chiropractors and physical therapists. But we treat the whole body, every structure and organ, and every patient is different. Even if I happen to see 10 people with back pain, each of those cases will be different. Their bodies are different, the cause of the pain is different, and their treatments will be different. Plus, my patients are much more diverse than that. I see newborns, toddlers, teenagers, desk workers, athletes, pregnant women – you name it. Everyone is a unique puzzle, and it's my job to uncover the clues and find the solution. It's a wonderful feeling being able to make people feel 'normal' again.

My advice to osteopathy students is to take your time choosing a specialty. Aim for general practice and get as much exposure as you can to the many aspects of this work."

PERSONAL QUALIFICATIONS

OSTEOPATHIC PHYSICIANS MUST have a very good bedside manner. Because many of their patients come to them with ailments that have been issues for a long time, there can be emotionally charged conversations that will take place. Being sick is quite stressful, and patients want to feel like their physician really understands them and their individual needs. Having a positive attitude is one of the most important personal qualifications for osteopathic physicians. All in all, you have to be the kind of person patients feel comfortable with when they are most vulnerable.

People pursuing careers in osteopathic medicine should also be innately curious. They should instinctively question why things are happening so they can get to the root of what is truly going on. Being inquisitive in this manner also helps them ask the patients the right questions. Getting the right information is essential to developing the proper diagnosis and treatment plan. People can be very private about their problems and that can become a problem in itself. It takes exceptional communications skills to get to the heart of the problem.

Osteopathic physicians should also be genuinely interested in people. As a physician, you will be face-to-face with patient after patient, getting to know them and their histories intimately. It is your job to help them, and it is hard to fake empathy. You must be genuinely keen on making people's lives better in order to succeed in this field.

You must excel in science, particularly biology, anatomy, and chemistry. Successful osteopathic physicians are deeply interested in these subjects. They are also excellent test takers and very book smart, able to master the disciplines as well as pass certifications and exams necessary to become licensed to practice medicine.

Because osteopaths approach healthcare from a more holistic viewpoint, all of the facets of human beings fascinate them in general. They have a passion for helping and healing people, and they are especially dedicated to the areas of wellness and wellbeing. An interest in nutrition is also necessary, as changing a patient's diet and understanding how food affects the body is one of the first ways an osteopath will try to heal a patient.

If you seem to have a general healing touch, being an osteopathic physician might be a good role for you. These practitioners simply have a natural way about them, something inside that makes others feel comfortable and comforted. People thrive when they are in their care.

ATTRACTIVE FEATURES

THERE ARE MANY POSITIVE REASONS to consider a career path as an osteopathic physician. Some of these include prestige, money, the chance to help people, the longevity and stability of the career, and the chance to become a lifelong learner. First and most commonly mentioned, is the personal gratification practitioners get from the work.

There is an air of prestige around being a physician. You are automatically well respected within your community simply for having the title "Doctor." You are seen as having accomplished something greater than most other individuals have or could ever dream of. You have made it through the trying years of medical school, and now you actually save lives as a career. As a physician, those you meet might even revere you. It is one of the few career paths where this is the case, where people are so impressed by what you are doing with your life that they automatically have a deep underlying respect for you.

Physicians are known for making excellent money. The starting salary for osteopaths is much higher than most jobs, and depending on the nature and success of your practice, it can rise to very high levels. If you work in higher income areas or with celebrities, you can charge higher rates.

Many doctors also love this career because they genuinely like to help people. They make a direct impact on society and people's lives. By becoming an osteopathic physician, you will be curing people's ailments and healing the sick. You will be able to relieve some of their emotional distress as well as their physical ailments, making it much more likely that their healing is permanent.

This is a stable career with an excellent outlook for the foreseeable future. There will never be a shortage of people who need help with their medical conditions. With the current Western lifestyle, our way of eating, our overwhelming work schedules, and our levels of stress, people are getting sicker than ever before. At the same time, the trend in healthcare is toward alternative and holistic methods. More and more people are becoming dissatisfied with traditional Western medicine and the reliance on pharmaceutical drugs, and are seeking out remedies that are more natural. This makes it a perfect time to become an osteopathic physician.

This is an attractive field for anyone who loves to learn. Osteopaths have to stay on top of the latest trends in health and wellness as well as the many different emerging technologies that heal. The most successful and satisfied osteopathic physicians are lifelong learners.

UNATTRACTIVE FEATURES

THIS IS ONE OF THE FEW FIELDS where you literally confront life and death situations.

Your patients are always your top priority, which can affect your own personal relationships, as well as hobbies, rest and relaxation. This can add an extra layer of stress. Being a physician is not just a job, it is a life commitment. If you want to lead a successful and happy life outside of the hospital or practice, you will need to surround yourself with very understanding and patient people – family and friends. Like it or not, you will probably end up disappointing people you care about from time to time.

Being a doctor also requires great sacrifices during the training phase. Your time will be spent studying non-stop, absorbing as much information as you can to prepare for passing tests and getting certifications. The human body has thousands of moving parts that all work together. It can seem like an overwhelming task to understand how each of them works, both separately and together. On top of that you have to consider environmental and outside factors that affect the human body. There is a massive amount of information to master.

There are certainly plenty of patients with common ailments you will immediately recognize and know just how to treat, but it is not always that easy. There will be patients presenting mysterious symptoms, diseases that will inexplicably not respond to treatment, and problems that will dumbfound you. It is your job to ferret out the details and get to the real cause of the problem. Sometimes this means trying a lengthy series of therapies that do not work, before finally coming up with some answers. This process can be a source of major frustration for both you and the patient.

Being a physician can also be emotionally taxing. Like it or not, some patients will have incurable issues. You will see people's health deteriorate before your eyes. You may form emotional attachments to your patients, and some of them will die. You might feel responsible, guilty, or even devastated. Every physician knows, at least intellectually, that it is impossible to save every patient. Still, it can be very hard to cope with the reality.

Perhaps the most obvious downside to becoming a physician of any kind, is the cost of medical school. While it is true that doctors make impressive incomes, they typically graduate from medical school with a mountain of debt. Even with incomes of six figures, it can take years to pay off the student loans.

EDUCATION AND TRAINING

OBTAINING A CAREER IN MEDICINE requires a long period of education and training. It first begins in high school with achieving high enough grades to get into a respected college or university.

An osteopathic physician in training will need to attend a four-year undergraduate program and obtain a bachelor's degree in an area that has a strong scientific background. Options like biology, chemistry, or neuroscience, are the popular choices for an undergraduate degree in this field. While a Bachelor of Science degree is not technically required for admission into medical school, having one will significantly improve your chances. Studies during the four years of undergraduate work will be concentrated on learning:

Anatomy, the make-up of the human body including

skeletal and muscular systems

Pathology, cells and pathogens like bacteria and viruses and their effect on their host

Biology, the genetic make-up of life

Chemistry, the fundamental building blogs of our universe

Organic Chemistry, deciphering the workings of living cells

After earning a bachelor's degree, the next step is to apply to medical school. Medical school admissions officers look closely at undergraduate grades, the particular degree program, and MCAT (Medical College Admission Test) scores. The MCAT is a required standardized test that will evaluate the applicant's knowledge in areas that are relevant to the field of medicine. It is a five-hour computerized test that covers physical science, chemistry, biology, critical thinking, verbal skills, and writing abilities.

Prospective osteopaths attend medical schools that specialize in osteopathic medicine. DO and MD medical programs have more similarities than differences. Both programs require an undergraduate degree and basic science coursework before admission. Both are typically four years in length, with two years of traditional science coursework and two years of clinical rotations. Both degrees will also prepare you to work as a fully-licensed physician in any medical specialty.

There are some key differences, however. Osteopathic programs have a strong emphasis on primary care with the focus on promoting a holistic, preventive approach to health. In addition, osteopathic medical students receive additional training in osteopathic manipulative treatment (OMT), which is using hands to diagnose and treat illness.

Osteopathic medical schools do not have an affiliated teaching hospital. Unlike traditional medical schools, they partner with medical facilities and physicians' offices in their local community. The advantage to this approach is it offers students the opportunity to learn in a variety of settings. However, it does not offer early exposure to research, cutting-edge treatments, or the kind of hands-on instruction one would expect to find in a traditional teaching hospital. There are some opportunities for research in osteopathic medicine, but students who are preparing for a career in medical research will find more opportunities as an MD.

In addition to over 500 osteopathic residency programs, osteopathic physicians have the option of entering the National Residency Matching Program, the same residency-matching program as MDs. The residency is entirely focused on in-hospital training instead of in-classroom experience. The length of the residency depends on the area of specialty, but the process typically takes three to seven years in total, following graduation from medical school.

In the first year, residents sit for the medical licensing examination. After completing the residency, they have the option to continue on with a general post-residency fellowship or focus on a more specialized area.

Every osteopath needs a license to practice medicine. Every state has different rules and requirements. Typical requirements include completion of at least a one-year residency. Most doctors choose to take it further and obtain the voluntary board certification. This certification confirms that the doctor has been tested in knowledge and skills, and is fully qualified to practice in a specialty. Certifications are renewed after a period of no less than six years. Some states also require doctors to take a certain number of hours of continuing medical education to ensure that they remain current on best practices.

EARNINGS

PHYSICIANS ARE WIDELY RECOGNIZED as having one of the highest salary ranges of all careers. However, when considering salary, you must take into account the amount of money spent on medical school education. Many doctors will be working their way out of that student debt burden for a long time to come before they actually see a healthy return on their investment. With rising healthcare costs and diminished reimbursements from health insurance companies, doctors in some cases are making less money than you would expect.

Earnings for physicians are dependent on a number of factors including geographic location and cost of living. Overall, most physicians earn incomes of between $175,000 and $200,000 in the United States. While osteopaths have some of the highest salaries possible in medicine, many osteopaths have salaries of $150,000 per year on average. The highest paying states for osteopathic physicians specifically are Washington (almost $300,000 per year), Arizona ($185,000), California ($180,000), New Jersey ($130,000), Ohio ($140,000), and Pennsylvania ($110,000).

Generally, the more experience an osteopath has, the higher the salary. In fact, some osteopaths who have been in practice for more than 10 years enjoy salaries of $300,000 all the way up to $500,000.

An osteopathic physician's salary also depends on the type of employer. For example, an osteopath employed by a hospital might be paid $150,000 per year, while an osteopathic physician in a private practice could expect to see a bit more at about $170,000. Self-employed osteopaths average around $200,000, but that high income can be misleading. Any self-employed professional has to account for additional taxes, insurance, cost of benefits, and overhead, and for doctors, malpractice insurance.

Much of what determines an osteopath's salary is the particular specialty. For example, an osteopath who focuses on radiology has a high median salary of $275,000 while an osteopath who specializes in the area of pediatrics receives only about $150,000 per year. Other specialties are paid annually as follows:

- Surgery
  $250,000

- Internal medicine
  $160,000

- Psychiatry
  $165,000

- Oncology
  $235,000

- Neurology
  $180,000

- OB-GYN
  $220,000

OPPORTUNITIES

ACCORDING TO THE AMERICAN Association of Colleges of Osteopathic Medicine, the United States is about to see an unprecedented shortage of physicians. There could be a critical gap of between 50,000 and 100,000 fewer physicians than are needed nationwide! The increasing need for physicians is commonly attributed to a rise in diseases like cancer and diabetes, the growing obesity rate, Baby Boomers reaching retirement age, increasing levels of air pollution, and people eating more unhealthy foods. The medical profession is having a difficult time keeping up with the demand and currently, there are not enough medical school graduates to fill the need. The good news is the resulting job outlook is great for future osteopaths.

Interestingly, there are more osteopaths entering the workforce than MDs. There is currently an average of 4,200 osteopathic physicians starting practice every year. Only seven percent of currently practicing doctors are osteopathic physicians, but more than 20 percent of physicians in training are choosing the career path of osteopathic medicine. The nation has approximately 63,000 fully licensed osteopathic physicians who practice today in various specialties.

There is further evidence that osteopathic medicine is a growing field with plenty of opportunity. The number of colleges that specialize in osteopathic medicine in the United States is increasing. Currently, there are 30 colleges of osteopathic medicine and four branch campuses, but there are several new osteopathic colleges in the planning stages that are expected to begin admitting students in the next few years.

More patients than ever are seeking out osteopathic physicians to treat their ailments because traditional Western medicine has not worked for them. There has been an increase in awareness of more holistic healthcare. Americans are becoming increasingly suspicious of pharmaceutical drugs, corporate farming, industrial pollutants, processed foods, and the stressful Western lifestyle in general. It is only natural that they also would become similarly interested in health and wellness, and specifically, the holistic approach to it practiced by osteopathic physicians.

GETTING STARTED

LONG BEFORE YOU GRADUATE FROM college you should start laying the groundwork for your career. Start by considering your options. What specialty interests you? Where do you want to practice? Do you want to be a staff doctor employed by a hospital, or go into private practice? Take the time to investigate your options, do your homework, and talk to as many people as you can.

When choosing a specialty, consider not only what interests you, but also what is most in demand. For example, family practice is very promising right now. There are more jobs available than physicians to fill them. With certification in family practice, you will literally be able to pick and choose among multiple offers and packages.

Internships and other forms of hands-on clinical practice will be an important part of your education. Stay on the lookout for chances to volunteer. Community service organizations, community health centers, and nursing homes are just a few of the places that usually need additional help.

Make sure your supervisors know that you are excited about your career choice. Always strive to go above and beyond what is asked of you and take on extra responsibilities. It is a subtle form of self-promotion that will pay off in the end.

Networking is important in this career. Attend seminars at your school, healthcare conferences, workshops, and any other activity where osteopaths gather. Even small meetings provide a special opportunity to interact with established professionals. There are usually question and answer sessions following these kinds of events. Make sure you take advantage of this time to ask questions, clarify issues you might have, or open up topics that may be new to you. It is a good way to sharpen your communications skills while making valuable contacts.

Networking is the best way to get your first job, but there are several other good ways to get started. Your college placement center will have listings of job openings. Check with your department head, too. It is common for research centers, clinics, and hospitals to have relationships with faculty members. Opportunities are often filled from the inside without ever being advertised or listed on a job board.

Join professional associations such as the American Osteopathic Association and the Student Osteopathic Medical Association. Do not overlook the associations for individual specialties, such as the American Osteopathic Academy of Sports Medicine or the Osteopathic Family Physician. Most osteopaths belong to more than one. Actively participate. Attend meetings, join committees, and interact socially. It is the best way to eventually meet just about everyone within your field. Like most medical niches, osteopathic medicine is a small universe with a finite number of people involved. The sooner you meet them, the better, because they will be your colleagues for many years to come. Professional associations also maintain job boards and advertise openings in their journals.

There are employment agencies that specialize in healthcare jobs, both on the Internet and off. You can apply directly to potential employers such as hospitals, clinics, and private medical practices. You may find it is more expedient to connect with a few good recruiters. If you are in a hurry to get work, sign on with a locum company. DOs who work as locum tenens report that they seldom go without work for longer than a week.

ASSOCIATIONS

■ American Association of American Colleges of Osteopathic Medicine (AACOM)
http://www.aacom.org

■ American Osteopathic Association (AOA)
http://www.osteopathic.org

■ Student Osteopathic Medical Association (SOMA)
https://www.studentdo.com

■ American Academy of Osteopathy
https://netforum.avectra.com/eweb/StartPage.aspx?Site=AAO

■ American Osteopathic Academy of Sports Medicine
www.aoasm.org/index.cfm

■ American Academy of Osteopathic Physicians
https://www.acoi.org

■ American Academy of Osteopathic Internists
https://www.acoi.org

■ Osteopathic Family Physician
http://www.osteopathicfamilyphysician.org

PERIODICAL

■ Journal of Osteopathic Medicine
www.journalofosteopathicmedicine.com

WEBSITE

■ The Student Doctor Network
http://www.studentdoctor.net/do

Institute For Career Research

Website www.careers-internet.org

For information on other Careers Reports please contact

service@careers-internet.org